The
# Pregnancy Puzzle Book

*The Pregnancy Puzzle Book*
Fun & Games to Get You Through the Whole 9 Months

© The Ivy Press

**Seal Press**
Published by Seal Press
A Member of the Perseus Books Group
1700 Fourth Street
Berkeley, California
www.sealpress.com

Library of Congress Cataloging-in-Publication Data

The pregnancy puzzle book : fun and games to get you through the whole nine months / by Ivy Press.
pages cm
ISBN 978-1-58005-510-9 (pbk.)
1. Exercise for pregnant women. 2. Pregnant women—Health and hygiene. 3. Prenatal care. 4. Puzzles—Health aspects. 5. Games—Health aspects I. Ivy Press.
RG558.7.P74 2013
618.2'44—dc23
2013016153

9 8 7 6 5 4 3 2 1

Cover & interior design by Kate Basart/Union Pageworks
Printed in China
Distributed by Publishers Group West

# The Pregnancy Puzzle Book

## Fun & Games to Get You Through the Whole 9 Months

*Puzzles devised by Erica Budge*

SEAL PRESS

# introduction

Welcome to the *Pregnancy Puzzle Book*, the first of its kind to have puzzles that get shorter or simpler as they go along to suit your burgeoning Baby Brain.

A full-term pregnancy is reckoned to be 40 weeks. During Week Zero, "Preconception," you're having your period—the last for quite a few months, if all goes to plan. A few days later, you'll ovulate, conceive, and after that it's the fascinating process of growth and development, until at the end of Week 40 (or thereabouts) your baby is born. In this book, we've provided preconception puzzles for Week Zero, just to get you in the mood, followed by puzzles for every week of your pregnancy. You can start at this point when your pregnancy is confirmed and go back to the earlier weeks.

There are four sections of increasing simplicity. The first three cover the three trimesters and feature questions that fit the standard pregnancy development pattern, while the fourth section might help pass the tedious hours in the delivery room or at home. The final set of puzzles is intended to complement your first few weeks with your new baby boy or girl.

*Here are some of the kinds of pregnancy-themed word puzzles you can expect when you are expecting.*

* **Wordsearch:** find words hidden vertically, horizontally, diagonally, backwards, or forwards in a grid.

* **Crosswords:** both cryptic and quick.

* **Word dial:** make words of three or more letters always using the letter in the center, and avoiding plurals, proper names, and third person singular present tense verb forms; fewer letters are provided as you go along.

* **In other words:** anagrams.

* **Puzzler:** say what you see.

* **Enigma variations:** code puzzles.

* **What comes next?:** find the next element in the sequence.

* **In opposition:** words that mean the opposite of the given word.

* **Same old, same old:** words that mean the same as the given word.

* **Twin up:** make pairs out of groups of words.

* **Sort and shift:** sort words into categories of three.

* **Odd one out:** spot the imposter.

* **Call my bluff:** spot the correct definition.

* **Word in the middle:** find a word that can end one word and start another.

* **Word sandwich:** find a word that means the same as the word on either side of it.

* **Word chain:** change one word to another, altering one letter at a time in as few steps as possible.

* **Soundalikes:** words that sound the same but mean something different.

* **What is not:** words that don't belong in a group.

* **Wordplay:** make as many words as you can using only the letters in the phrase provided.

Plus a few random riddles and conundrums.

# 🐦 first trimester

## Congratulations! Assuming the thin blue line is correct and there are no complications, you are going to have a baby.

During the first trimester (the first 12 weeks) you may have nothing to show for this (except morning sickness, mood swings, headaches, total fatigue, and acne), but inside your uterus it is all systems go. This is a crucial time for your baby's development and your body is pumping out hormones and extra blood cells to make it happen. By the end of this trimester your baby will have gone from a microscopic mulberry-shaped dot to a perfectly formed little person about as long as your thumb.

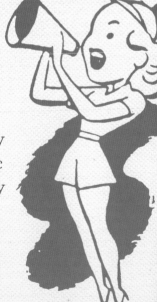

Scientists may poo-poo the idea of Baby Brain, but we can only assume they have never had a baby. Gradually you will realize that there are some life events the smarter parts of the brain just can't handle, and that they should be quiet and make space for the rest of the brain to do its job. However, that's not going to happen for a bit, so the first trimester puzzles are pretty much what you might expect for a non-pregnant solver. They have been conceived and designed to be done in short bursts between naps and to distract you from feeling too nauseous.

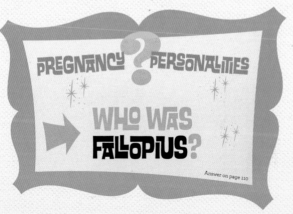

PREGNANCY? PERSONALITIES

WHO WAS FALLOPIUS?

Answer on page 110

# preconception

### 1. Word in the middle

What word can be added to the end of the word on the left of the parentheses and the beginning of the word on the right of the parentheses to make two new phrases?

SLOW ( _MOTION_ ) SICKNESS

### 2. In other words

Unscramble the anagram:

PRANCE IN TO COT

### 3. Odd one out

Which is the odd word out?

BOTTLE          ONESIE          – CARRIER
STROLLER        – MITTENS        RATTLE

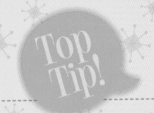

These puzzles will help limber up your brain for when you are pregnant—and welcome to all you puzzlers redirected from Week 4.

## 4. Word dial

Make as many words as you can of three letters or more, always including the central letter. Give yourself an extra point for making a word out of all the letters.

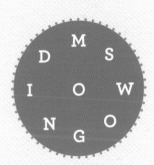

*DOG*
*MOW*
*SOW*
*NOW*
*GOD*
*mowing*
*sowing*

## 5. Same old, same old

Which word means the same as to "twitch" or "irritate"?

VACILLATE    VENTILATE    VERMICULATE
VELLICATE    VITIATE    VITUPERATE

# week one

6. ## Word in the middle

What word can be added to the end of the word on the left of the parentheses and the beginning of the word on the right of the parentheses to make two new phrases?

PELVIC ( _ _ _ _ _ ) POLISH

7. ## Sort and shift

Sort these 12 words into four categories of three:

TEDDY          BALL           TRIANGLE
NET            TAMBOURINE     POLYGON
CIRCLE         RATTLE         MARACA
RACKET         SQUARE         BLOCKS

| | | | |
|---|---|---|---|
| 1 | | | |
| 2 | | | |
| 3 | | | |
| 4 | | | |

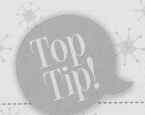

It's now one week after your period, and your uterus is getting ready for a guest. Now it's up to Egg and Sperm to do their best.

8. ## Odd one out

Which is the odd word out?

REFBER       PKAR       RIKK
REASS        OSKPC      ARAGP

9. ## Enigma variations

What six letters are missing on the fourth line of this code?

TTLS
HIWWYA
UATWSH
——————
TTLS
HIWWYA

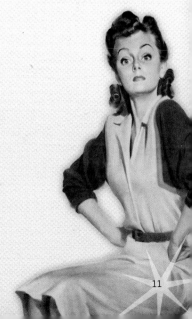

# week two

### 10. Word chain

Your baby is currently a mass of multiplying cells that looks a bit like a mulberry. Silkworms feed on mulberry trees. Can you get from "worm" to "silk" in six steps?

WORM _____ _____ _____ _____ _____ SILK

### 11. Word dial

Make as many words as you can of three letters or more, always including the central letter. Give yourself an extra point for making a word out of all the letters.

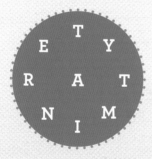

Your fertilized egg, multiplying as it goes, is now bowling down the Fallopian tube towards the uterus and implantation.

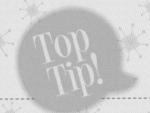

**Top Tip!**

## 12. Same old, same old

Which word means the same as "burping"?

EXPATIATION    ESCAPEMENT    ERUCTATION
EXTIRPATION    EPILATION    EXHORTATION

## 13. In other words

Unscramble the anagram:

SUTURE

## 14. Word in the middle

What word can be added to the end of the word on the left of the parentheses and the beginning of the word on the right of the parentheses to make two new phrases?

FERTILIZED ( EGG ) TIMER

# week three

### 15. Word in the middle

What word can be added to the end of the word on the left of the parentheses and the beginning of the word on the right of the parentheses to make two new phrases?

**HEAVY (_____) FATIGUE**

### 16. Same old, same old

Which word means the same as "peeing"?

**MACHICOLATION**          **MASTICATION**

**MALDISTRIBUTION**        **MENSURATION**

**MICTURITION**            **MORIGERATION**

### 17. In other words

Unscramble the anagram:

**DEB STATUS**

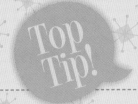

You may feel suddenly exhausted, or get a strange metallic taste in your mouth. Don't worry, this is totally normal.

18. ## Word dial

Make as many words as you can of three letters or more, always including the central letter. Give yourself an extra point for making a word out of all the letters.

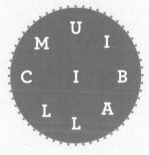

19. ## Call my bluff

What does "nictitation" mean?

Swimming at night

Meditating on the futility of existence

Rapid or excessive blinking

A Scottish legal term

Adulterating alcoholic drinks

# week four

## 20. Linked in

What one word links these words?

BIRD        CALL        FISH
SCRATCH    POUNCE    LITTER
MOUSE       NAP         WALK

## 21. Word chain

Can you get from "wind" to "calm" in six steps?

WIND \_\_\_\_\_ \_\_\_\_\_ \_\_\_\_\_ \_\_\_\_\_ \_\_\_\_\_CALM

## 22. In other words

Unscramble the anagram:

FOIL A PLAN

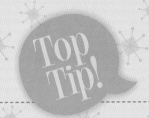
The thin blue line says you really are pregnant. If you haven't done the first few pages of puzzles already, go back and start with week zero.

## 23. Wordsearch

You need your vitamins. Find 18 fruity words hidden in this wordsearch. The words run horizontally, vertically, or diagonally, and may go backwards or forwards. Some words may share a letter.

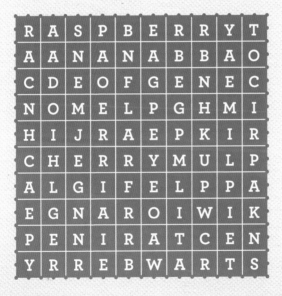

| R | A | S | P | B | E | R | R | Y | T |
|---|---|---|---|---|---|---|---|---|---|
| A | A | N | A | N | A | B | B | A | O |
| C | D | E | O | F | G | E | N | E | C |
| N | O | M | E | L | P | G | H | M | I |
| H | I | J | R | A | E | P | K | I | R |
| C | H | E | R | R | Y | M | U | L | P |
| A | L | G | I | F | E | L | P | P | A |
| E | G | N | A | R | O | I | W | I | K |
| P | E | N | I | R | A | T | C | E | N |
| Y | R | R | E | B | W | A | R | T | S |

# week five

### 24. What is not?

Right now, your embryo is the size of an apple seed. Which of these is not a variety of apple?

ANANAS REINETTE
WINTER PEARMAIN
LARKSPUR FERDINAND
BEDFORDSHIRE FOUNDLING
DOUBLE RED JONATHAN
KNOBBED RUSSET

### 25. Odd one out

As well as being the size of an apple seed, your embryo is also pear-shaped. Which is the odd one out in the following list of pear varieties?

| | | |
|---|---|---|
| ANJOU | BARTLETT | COMICE |
| PACKHAM | ROCHA | WILLIAMS |

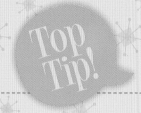

You may want to look at your caffeine intake. Most doctors recommend no more than one mug of coffee a day.

## 26. Sort and shift

Sort the following 12 words into four categories:

CREAM      JUG        CHOCOLATE
LEMON      COFFEE     TEA
SUGAR      POT        HONEY
CUP        MILK       MOLASSES

| 1 | | | |
|---|---|---|---|
| 2 | | | |
| 3 | | | |
| 4 | | | |

## 27. What is not?

Which one of these is not a kind of tea?

ROSE POUCHONG          FUJI MITSU
ORANGE PEKOE           LAPSANG SOUCHONG
GYOKURO                SENCHA FUKUYU

# week six

## 28. Cryptic crossword

In a cryptic crossword, the clue is a word puzzle in and of itself. Don't get stuck on a surface reading—wordplay is part of the game. Embedded words, double definitions, anagrams, and reversals are a few of the tricky twisters so keep your eyes peeled.

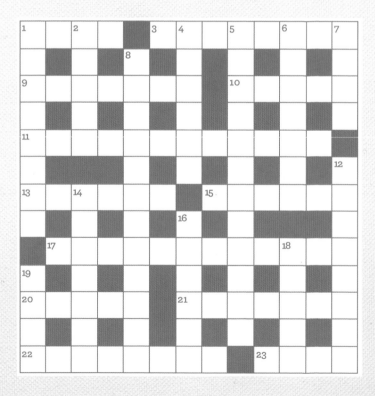

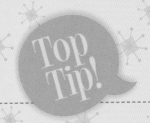

## Across

1. Choose the best (4)
3. Can't leap wildly after birth (8)
9. Kind of exercise I, Bo, care about (7)
10. Never confuse courage and audacity (5)
11. Lacking 10 across, I fear that den terribly (5-7)
13. Fame from being up tree in mess (6)
15. Rob, confused has a look in: he does what he's told (6)
17. It lies in bed with gravity, and is not good to eat (12)
20. Bail? I would be doubtful with such a plea (5)
21, 22. Complaint of pregnancy sounds like grieving illness (7, 8)
23. Nothing found in bronze room (4)

## Down

1. Stage of farm plot development (8)
2. Soldier follows company recruitment head, the dog (5)
4. A bit of hair on Queen Elizabeth is in the cupboard (6)
5. Playing a part in country, or bit, anyhow (12)
6. Room for a child to care for the railway (7)
7. Getting on with the heads of all gynecological education departments (4)
8. Pregnancy specialist: "I bet I can sort problem" (12)
12. Notes on a soft egg implanted in Rio (8)
14. Quiet action moves the car (7)
16. Layer of skin found in bladder mishap (6)
18. Be rid of problems—she's getting married (5)
19. Go by the canyon and succeed (4)

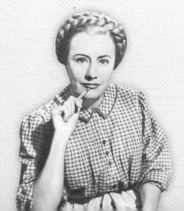

# week seven

## 29. Twin up

Your uterus is now the size of a tennis ball. Pair up these 16 words to make eight tennis-related terms:

TENNIS     BALL     MATCH

FOOT     MIXED     SECOND

GRAND     LINE     FAULT

BOY     POINT     SLAM

DOUBLES     COACH     JUDGE

SERVICE

## 30. Enigma variations

Your embryo's heart now beats twice as fast as yours. What's wrong with the sentence below?

A

BIRD IN THE

THE HAND IS WORTH

TWO IN THE BUSH

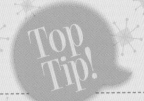
Your clothes will begin to get a bit tight as your uterus jostles for space with your other internal organs. Time for a new wardrobe!

## 31. Word sandwich

Place a word in the parentheses that means the same as the words on either side of the parentheses:

Break out of your shell (_____) useful hole in a wall

## 32. In opposition

What is the opposite of "flammable"?

INFLAMMABLE          FIREPROOF
BURNABLE             INEFFABLE
INCANDESCENT         DAMP

## 33. In other words

Unscramble the anagram:

I AM IN COT

# week eight

### 34. Soundalikes

You may be offered your first ultrasound scan around now. Below are paired definitions that will lead you to words that sound alike but are spelled differently and mean different things.

What you breathe/the receiver of your fortune

A refreshing alcoholic beverage/that which carries you off

An ominous noise/a watery byway

Modest and unremarkable/completely separate

To get in exchange for effort/it holds lots of tea

The basis of bread/the basis of a bunch

### 35. Word sandwich

Place a word in the parentheses that means the same as the two words on either side of the parentheses:

BLOW UP (_____) REALLY GREAT

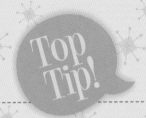
## 36. In opposition

If anyone has guessed, or you have told everyone, you may be fed up with well-meaning advice and wish everyone would just be quiet. What is the opposite of "taciturn"?

CONVIVIAL     GREGARIOUS     GARRULOUS

VIVACIOUS     EMOTIONAL

## 37. What is not?

Your embryo is about the size of a small olive. Which of these is not an olive?

KALAMATA     MANZANILLA

PICHOLINE     LUGANO

TEMPRANILLO     SEVILLANO

## 38. Wordsearch

Find 14 scent-related words in this grid. Words may run horizontally, vertically or diagonally, backwards, and forwards. Some words may share a letter.

| G | R | E | P | I | N | U | J | T | D |
|---|---|---|---|---|---|---|---|---|---|
| R | N | R | K | S | U | M | R | O | E |
| E | A | A | M | B | E | R | O | M | N |
| V | B | D | L | C | D | W | S | A | I |
| I | E | E | F | Y | L | G | E | G | M |
| T | H | C | I | A | G | J | K | R | S |
| E | L | M | D | P | I | N | E | E | A |
| V | A | N | I | L | L | A | A | B | J |
| N | A | O | P | N | E | R | O | L | I |
| S | R | E | D | N | E | V | A | L | Y |

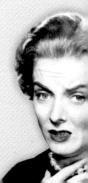

26

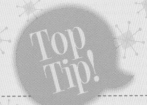
Top Tip!

The smell of certain foods or other people's perfume can make you nauseous. A sniff of a slice of ginger may help.

## 39. Linked in

What word links these words?

PUMP            LOCK            CRAFT
FRAME           BAG             LIFT
HEAD            GUITAR

## 40. Word chain

Hold your nose and get from "scent" to "stink" in three steps:

SCENT     _____  _____     STINK

## 41. Word in the middle

What word can be added to the end of the word on the left of the parentheses and the beginning of the word on the right of the parentheses to make two new phrases?

NASAL (_____) FEED

# week ten

## 42. What is not?

Your embryo—now officially a fetus—is bigger than a large grape. Which of the following is not a grape variety?

BARBERA               GEWÜRZTRAMINER
NEBBIOLO              PINOTAGE
VIONNET               ZINFANDEL

## 43. Sort and shift

Sort the following 15 words into five categories:

| RED | RED | RED | YELLOW |
|-----|-----|-----|--------|
| YELLOW | YELLOW | BLUE | BLUE |
| BLUE | GREEN | GREEN | PURPLE |
| PURPLE | ORANGE | ORANGE | |

| | | | | |
|---|---|---|---|---|
| 1 | | | | |
| 2 | | | | |
| 3 | | | | |
| 4 | | | | |
| 5 | | | | |

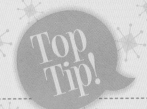

Top Tip!

Your blood volume will increase up to 40 percent as your fetus grows, so help out by drinking plenty of water.

## 44. In opposition

What is the opposite of "deliquesce"?

UNIFY      SOLIDIFY      THICKEN
COAGULATE      EMULSIFY      EVAPORATE

## 45. In other words

Unscramble the anagram:

DIRTY NOAH

## 46. Same old, same old

Which word means the same as "sleep inducing"?

SOMNAMBULANT      SOLANACEAE
SOPORIFIC      SOMNOLENT
SOMBROUS      SOPHOMORIC

# week eleven

### 47. **Word dial**

Make as many words as you can of three or more letters, always including the central letter. Give yourself an extra point for making a word out of all the letters.

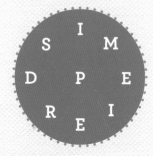

### 48. **Odd one out**

Your fetus is now the size of a small apple. Pick the bad apple out of the following list:

BASE            ATE             PAMPHLET
MENTAL          FARMER          LADDER
RAREST          STAPLE

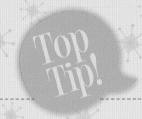

Your first outbreak of acne since your teens; blame your hormones, and make yourself an oatmeal face mask.

## 49. Call my bluff

What does "thiamine" mean?

A vibrating musical instrument

Having a slightly underfunctioning thyroid gland

A sulphur-based water-soluble vitamin of the B complex

Relating to the dialect found on the smaller Pacific islands

Bluish lead-based pigment used by pre-Renaissance artists

Having very slender thighs

## 50. In other words

Unscramble the anagram:

NINE MOIST ACES

# week twelve

### 51. In other words

Unscramble the anagram:

**A TURNIP RIOT**

### 52. Word chain

You might find you are slobbering a bit due to morning sickness. Can you get from "spit" to "lick" in six steps?

**SPIT** _____ _____ _____ _____ _____ **LICK**

### 53. Word dial

Make as many words as you can of three or more letters, always including the central letter. Give yourself an extra point for making a word out of all the letters.

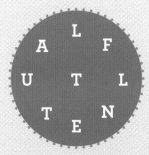

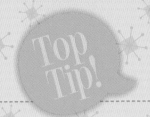

You will be in the grip of titanic mood swings. It is all hormones, you can explain later, although your mommy friends may already guess what's up.

## 54. Enigma variations

What is the missing word?

ROUND    SWISH    BEEP    ___    SHH

## 55. Call my bluff

Hormones are affecting your nose, causing congestion and other troubles. What does "epistaxis" mean?

Ancient Greek philosopher of the school of Parmenides

A genus of foul-smelling shrub from South America

A figure of speech in which too many words are used to describe an object

Medical term for nosebleed

A state of total boredom

The atrophied claw on a possum's back foot

You have passed the three-month mark and weathered the morning sickness and the constant fatigue. You have also finished the first set of puzzles. Here is a quick review of progress so far, plus a fun pregnancy quiz.

- Your baby now has all the major organs in place and a recognizable face, with a nose, eyelids, ears and the beginnings of lips.

- He or she is about 3 inches long. Brain and muscles are beginning to hook up. The baby has opposable thumbs and can kick, swallow, and hiccup.

- You can start eating three snacks a day in between your three main meals, as long as they are not chips or chocolate.

- You can start telling everyone your news if you haven't already, as the chance of a miscarriage is significantly lowered.

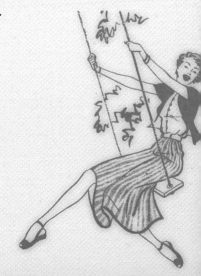

# first trimester pregnancy quiz

1. When does a zygote become an embryo? And when does an embryo become a fetus?

2. What is the "pregnancy hormone" and where is it produced?

3. What chromosome is required to produce a boy, and who provides it?

4. What chromosome is required to produce a girl, and who provides it?

5. Why is folic acid essential in your diet in the first trimester?

6. How much weight should an average-sized woman gain during pregnancy?

7. How many extra calories per day does a pregnant woman need for optimum health?

8. What percentage of pregnant women report morning sickness in the first trimester?

9. Which of your baby's organs developed first?

10. How much liquid should you be drinking each day?

# second trimester

Hooray! You have made it to the calm waters of the second trimester, and are now officially in the radiant and blooming period, although it may not always feel like that.

During the second trimester (13–27 weeks) you move from looking a bit chunky to a proper pregnancy shape (which can vary a great deal) with a definite bump. Your baby spends most of this period growing longer and larger, finishing off any organ formation left over from the first trimester and finessing the details such as toenails and eyelashes. He or she will also start moving, often at night. Regard being constantly woken as practice for the weeks after the birth.

Now that you are in the calm stage, the puzzles have been adjusted to suit your needs. Serious Baby Brain kicks in around Week 23, when you find that you forget little things instantly (because they don't really matter) or lose focus very easily (because your baby is River Dancing its way around your uterus). To help you, more clues have been introduced in this section, and the puzzles are designed to suit a diminished attention span, becoming either shorter or simpler. This makes them an ideal diversion when you are waiting to be called in for your next ultrasound scan, or for short bursts between naps.

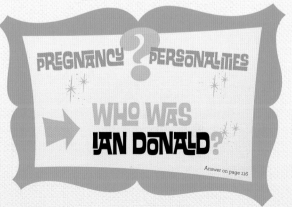

PREGNANCY ? PERSONALITIES

WHO WAS
IAN DONALD?

Answer on page 116

# week thirteen

### 56. Word dial

Make as many words as you can of three or more letters, always including the central letter. Give yourself an extra point for making a word out of all the letters.

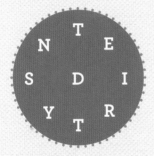

### 57. Odd one out

Most of your baby's organs are now fully formed. Find the odd one out from this list:

| | | |
|---|---|---|
| LIVER | SKIN | KIDNEY |
| HEART | LUNGS | BRAIN |
| ULNA | STOMACH | INTESTINE |

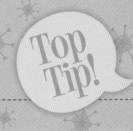

**Top Tip!** Get your teeth and gums checked out; pregnancy hormones make gums ultra sensitive and vulnerable.

## 58. Linked in

What word links these words?

| | | |
|---|---|---|
| COMB | DOG | EGG |
| ENAMEL | EYE | FAIRY |
| PICK | SABER | SAW |

## 59. Word sandwich

Place a word in the parentheses that means the same as the two words outside the parentheses:

PRACTICE (_ _ _ _ _ _) TOOL

## 60. In other words

Unscramble the anagram:

SHOUT WHAM

# week fourteen

### 61. Wordsearch

Your baby is now growing lots of hair. Find 15 hair-related words in this wordsearch. Words may run horizontally, vertically, diagonally, backwards, or forwards. Some letters may appear in more than one word.

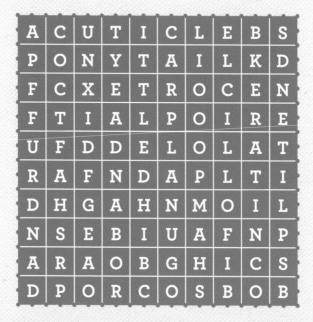

| A | C | U | T | I | C | L | E | B | S |
|---|---|---|---|---|---|---|---|---|---|
| P | O | N | Y | T | A | I | L | K | D |
| F | C | X | E | T | R | O | C | E | N |
| F | T | I | A | L | P | O | I | R | E |
| U | F | D | D | E | L | O | L | A | T |
| R | A | F | N | D | A | P | L | T | I |
| D | H | G | A | H | N | M | O | I | L |
| N | S | E | B | I | U | A | F | N | P |
| A | R | A | O | B | G | H | I | C | S |
| D | P | O | R | C | O | S | B | O | B |

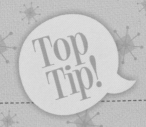

**Top Tip!**

Your baby's gender is now established; decide before your next ultrasound if you want to know whether it's a boy or a girl.

## 62. Word chain

You may be a martyr to hemorrhoids right now. Can you get from "piles" to "balms" in three careful steps?

PILES  _____  _____  BALMS

## 63. Word sandwich

Your size requires comfy pants. Place a word in the parentheses that means the same as the two words outside the parentheses:

EXPAND (_____) JAIL TIME

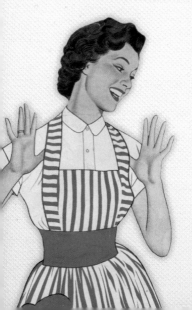

# week fifteen

### 64. Sort and shift

Sort the following nine words into three categories:

| DOOR | THIGH | JUGULAR |
|------|-------|---------|
| BREAST | HATCH | PORTAL |
| GATE | WING | FEMORAL |

|   |   |   |   |
|---|---|---|---|
| 1 |   |   |   |
| 2 |   |   |   |
| 3 |   |   |   |

### 65. Soundalikes

Identify the triple homonym:

Wind indicator

Full of unjustified self-regard

Part of the circulatory system

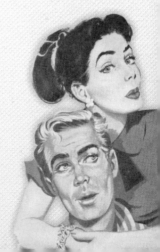

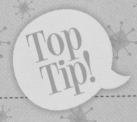

### 66. Call my bluff

The good news is your sex life has perked up. What does "jouissance" mean?

Concentrated essence of papaya

A rarely used fencing maneuver

Orgasmic bliss

A provençal salad dressing

An ancient property regulation in New Orleans

A feeling of inexplicable cheerfulness

### 67. Enigma variations

Your baby can now point his or her toes and pull faces. Fill in the missing letters in the list below:

TLPWTM
TLPSAH
TLPHRB
TLPHN
ATLPW___ATWH

# week sixteen

### 68. Wordplay

Your baby is now the size of an avocado. How many words of three or four letters can you make out of these words?

**AVOCADO PEAR**

### 69. Round robin

Work out which letter replaces the question mark:

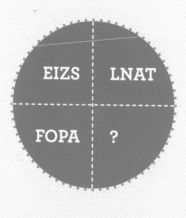

EIZS | LNAT

FOPA | ?

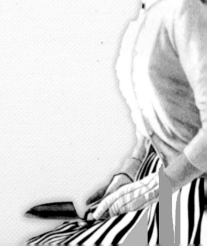

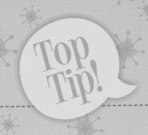

**Top Tip!**

Your baby can now suck his or her thumb; and so can you if you concentrate hard!

### 70. Word sandwich

Place a word in the brackets that means the same as the two words outside the brackets:

MAGPIE ( _ _ _ _ ) TYPE SIZE

### 71. What is not?

Which one of these is not a hormone?

ESTROGEN          FSH          PROGESTERONE
OXYTOCIN          HCG          TESTOSTERONE
THEOBROMINE

### 72. In other words

Unscramble the anagram:

THE URN BAR

# week seventeen

## 73. What comes next?

Your baby is now about 5 inches long and packs quite a punch. What comes next in this list?

FLY    BANTAM    LIGHT    WELTER    _ _ _ _ _ _?

## 74. What is not?

Your pelvis is beginning to feel the strain. Which one of these is not a bone in the pelvis?

ILIUM           COCCYX          ISTHMUS
SACRUM          ISCHIUM         PUBIS

## 75. Linked in

What word links these words?

DOG             COBRA           CAT
LOCUST          CAMEL           FISH
EAGLE           LION

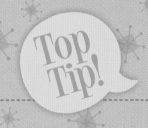

**Top Tip!**

Get up slowly—blood now takes longer to reach your upper body, leading to dizziness if you stand up too quickly.

### 76. In opposition

You need to pee more often as your cramped bladder fills up quicker. What is the opposite of "distended"?

EXTENDED     INFLATED     INTENDED

DEFLATED     CONTENDED     CONFLATED

### 77. Same old, same old

Which word means the same as "lower back pain"?

PLUMBAGO     LUMBRICUS     GALAGO

LUMBAGO     LUGANO     LANUGO

### 78. Puzzler

Solve the puzzler:

SPLIOACSNTE

# week eighteen

### 79. Soundalikes

Your baby can now hear sounds, including your voice. Below are trios of definitions that will lead you to words that sound alike but are spelled differently and mean different things.

Match/fruit/trim

Alternative/metal matrix/nautical implement

Precipitation/royal rule/control

Can be hard or soft/location/dress

### 80. Odd one out

Your baby now has 200 of his or her 206 bones. Which is the odd bone out?

| | | |
|---|---|---|
| TIBIA | FIBULA | FEMUR |
| ULNA | RADIUS | HUMERUS |

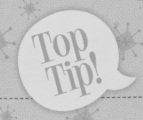

**Top Tip!**

To cure leg cramps at night, stand on a cold floor and lift your toes to stretch your calves.

### 81. **Word in the middle**

What word can be added to the end of the word on the left of the parentheses and the beginning of the word on the right of the parentheses to make two new phrases?

BLOOD (_____) HUG

### 82. **Word chain**

Can you go from "foot" to "shoe" in three easy steps?

FOOT _____ _____ SHOE

# week nineteen

### 83. Enigma variations

Work out these words in code to make names:

NBOPMP       CMBIMJL       DISJTUJBM

MPVCPVUJM     KJNNZ        DIPP

### 84. What comes next?

Your baby weighs at least 7 ounces. Based on that weight, what is the next letter?

G N ?

### 85. Word sandwich

Your baby's skin is still loose and wrinkly, like a baby elephant's. Place a word in the parentheses that means the same as the two words outside the parentheses:

SKIN (_____) CONCEAL

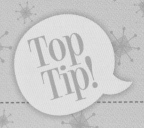

Your shoes feel tight as your feet and
ankles swell. Time to go shopping!

### 86. **What is not?**

Which of these is not part of the foot?

HALLUX     METATARSAL     TALUS
CALCANEUS     POLLEX

### 87. **Sort and shift**

Sort the following nine words into three categories:

BRAN     CHOP     FRET
LEND     MOST     TRAP
PART     SHED     WORD

1
2
3

# week twenty

## 88. Cryptic crossword

In a cryptic crossword, the clue is a word puzzle in and of itself. Don't get stuck on a surface reading—wordplay is part of the game. Embedded words, double definitions, anagrams, and reversals are a few of the tricky twisters so keep your eyes peeled.

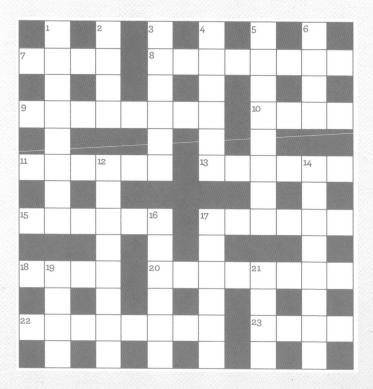

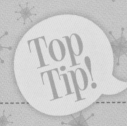

Time for your mid-pregnancy ultrasound. Take this crossword along in case you have to wait.

## Across

7. South American I can mix up (4)
8. The result of more than one pregnancy (8)
9. Invention—I care not wildly (8)
10. Does parts of a play (4)
11. Pair left in coupé (6)
13. In cubicle answer makes hygienic (6)
15. Meets Oriental back with respect (6)
17. Moving it back in the moon (6)
18. One of two children (4)
20. Alter man to make motherly (8)
22. She feeds the baby for you (3, 5)
23. Screening southern Canada briefly (4)

## Down

1. Change more on us—huge (8)
2. Pop art movement? (4)
3. Busy and animated (6)
4. Outdoor meal (6)
5. Can't Jade be moved near (8)
6. Try an exam (4)
12. Pen Grant is expecting (8)
14. Newborn disturbs Anne a lot (8)
16. My Rome recollection (6)
17. Look after a parent (6)
19. A question of time? (4)
21. The remainder relax (4)

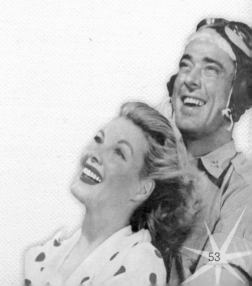

# week twenty-one

### 89. Word dial

Your baby is getting very active in the womb. Make as many words as you can of three letters or more, always including the central letter. Give yourself an extra point for making a word out of all the letters.

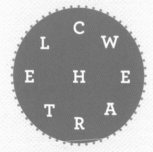

### 90. Puzzler

Decode the puzzler:

JACK

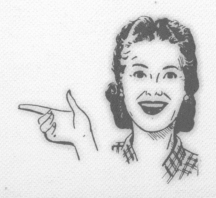

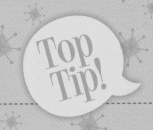

## 91. Call my bluff

Good food, tranquility, and gentle exercise can all help right now. What does "bidalasana" mean?

In yoga, the pose of the rabbit

An Indian dish of lentils and tamarind paste

In yoga, the pose of the dog

The state of being half-awake and half-asleep

In yoga, the pose of the cat

A mythical lake in Nepal

## 92. Same old, same old

Your navel may start to stick out, even if you have always had an "innie". Which word has the nearest meaning to "stick out" in this sense?

DETRUDE     EXTRUDE     EXUDE

INTRUDE     OBTRUDE     PROTRUDE

# week twenty-two

### 93. Word in the middle

What word can be added to the end of the word on the left of the parentheses and the beginning of the word on the right of the parentheses to make two new phrases?

BODY (_____) STROKE

### 94. In opposition

Your baby may wake at night and kick you awake, too. What is the opposite of insomnia?

HYPERSOMNIA    NARCOLEPSY    ASOMNIA

PARASOMNIA    DYSSOMNIA    SLEEP

### 95. Linked in

Your ligaments are relaxing, and your hips are achy. Take your mind off it by working out what word links these words:

SELL    SHELL    SOAP

TISSUE    TOUCH    WARE

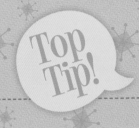

**Top Tip!**

Your body temperature is higher. Dress in layers so you can easily chill out when necessary.

## 96. Sort and shift

Your baby can now swallow and gulp. Sort the following nine words into three categories:

| PALM | GULP | NAIL |
| HANDSAW | HAWK | RASP |
| SWALLOW | SWIG | KNUCKLE |

| | | | |
|---|---|---|---|
| 1 | | | |
| 2 | | | |
| 3 | | | |

## 97. What is not?

Your uterus is now the size of a baseball holding its precious contents. Which of the following is not a recognized quality in a diamond?

| CUT | COLOR | CLARITY |
| CARAT | CONSISTENCY | |

### 98. Word dial

Make as many words as you can of three letters or more, always including the central letter. Give yourself an extra point for making a word out of all the letters.

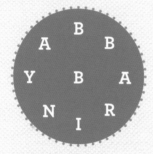

### 99. Same old, same old

Check your iron levels, as your baby is draining your blood bank. Which word means the same as "iron"?

**FERRUM**    **FERROUS**    **FERRET**
**FERRULE**    **FERAL**    **FERRY**

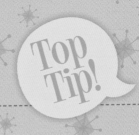

You forget unimportant stuff because you are focusing on more important priorities. Don't worry about it.

## 100. Twin up

Your baby is now about 12 inches long. Arrange these ten words into five pairs, each using one word from each box:

| ADMIRER | MARINES | DECIMAL | NIGHT | LARGE |
| --- | --- | --- | --- | --- |

| REGAL | CLAIMED | MARRIED | SEMINAR | THING |
| --- | --- | --- | --- | --- |

## 101. Word chain

Your little amnionaut is now bouncing around in the womb. Can you get from "moon" to "walk" in seven small steps?

MOON _____ _____ _____ _____ _____ _____ WALK

# week twenty-four

## 102. Same old, same old

Which word means the same as "the area around your nipple"?

**AURORA**              **AUREOLE**              **AREOLA**
**ARAGULA**             **AEOLIUS**              **ASTRAGALUS**

## 103. Enigma variations

Your baby is now viable and could possibly survive, with help, if born. Solve this puzzle:

**A plane crashed directly on the border between Canada and the USA. Where were the survivors buried?**

## 104. In other words

Unscramble the anagram:

**HORRID HOMES**

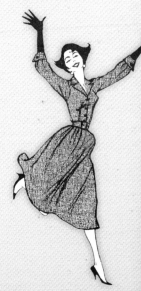

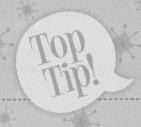

**Don't worry about your darkening nipples and face freckles; they will fade after birth.**

## 105. Wordsearch

Your baby spends a lot of time twirling around on the umbilical cord, rope dancing. Find 14 dance-related words in this wordsearch. Words may run horizontally, vertically, diagonally, backwards, or forwards. Some letters may appear in more than one word.

| G | I | J | A | C | B | J | I | V | E |
|---|---|---|---|---|---|---|---|---|---|
| C | A | K | L | O | P | D | E | E | L |
| T | R | F | G | R | H | D | I | B |   |
| E | J | U | K | E | L | N | M | N | O |
| U | O | P | M | C | A | O | A | Z | D |
| N | S | A | M | B | A | B | Q | T | O |
| I | R | S | A | T | A | M | U | L | S |
| M | E | R | E | N | G | U | E | A | A |
| S | A | L | S | A | V | K | S | W | P |
| S | X | Y | T | O | R | T | X | O | F |

# week twenty-five

## 106. In opposition

What is the opposite of "respiration"?

PERSPIRATION          INSPIRATION
EXHALATION            INHALATION
PHOTOSYNTHESIS

## 107. In other words

Time to start thinking about the big event. Unscramble the anagram:

PRINT BLAH

## 108. Linked in

Your baby can detect light. What word links these words?

BALL          BATH          BROW
LASH          LID           LINER
SHADOW        SOCKET        STRAIN

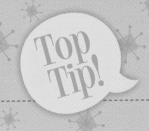

**Top Tip!**

You may find you are getting out of breath quickly as your lung capacity dwindles. Slow down.

## 109. Enigma variations

You may find spider veins on your breasts. They are nothing to worry about—they will eventually go away. Fill in the four missing letters below:

TIBS CUTWS
DCTR AWTSO
OCTS ADUATR
ATIBS _ _ _ _ _

## 110. Soundalikes

Your baby is putting on weight. What one word fits all these definitions?

An enclosure

To beat mercilessly

Unit of currency

Division of weight

A kind of cake

To throb or pulsate

# week twenty-six

### 111. Word dial

Your belly is now about the size of a medium beach ball, but not as light, and unfortunately you cannot just let the air out. Make as many words as you can of three letters or more, always including the central letter. Give yourself an extra point for making a word out of all the letters.

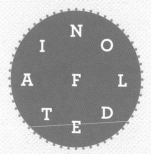

### 112. Word chain

Get from the left side to the other side in five steps:

LEFT \_\_\_\_ \_\_\_\_ \_\_\_\_ \_\_\_\_ SIDE

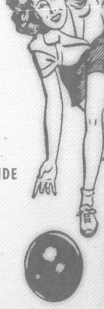

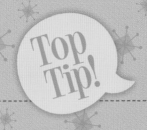

## 113. Word in the middle

What word can be added to the end of the word on the left of the parentheses and the beginning of the word on the right of the parentheses to make two new phrases?

BROAD (_ _ _ _) KICK

## 114. Odd one out

Your baby now weighs a little under 2 lbs. Which of these healthy foods is the odd one out?

BLUEBERRY    BROCCOLI    CABBAGE    CARROT
LETTUCE    PEPPER    STRAWBERRY  SPINACH

## 115. Linked in

Well over halfway through, and you may feel a bit down. What links these words?

ALICE    COBALT    ELECTRIC
NAVY    OXFORD    SKY

# week twenty-seven

## 116. Wordsearch

Time to take your mind off the pregnancy blues. Find 12 hobby-related words in this wordsearch. Words may run horizontally, vertically, diagonally, backwards, or forwards. Some letters may appear in more than one word.

| W | A | G | N | I | T | N | I | A | P |
|---|---|---|---|---|---|---|---|---|---|
| E | M | A | R | C | A | M | B | A | O |
| A | G | C | D | E | A | E | T | R | T |
| V | F | N | G | H | C | D | E | T |
| I | I | J | I | K | H | N | R | A | E |
| N | L | R | M | W | N | A | A | D | R |
| G | O | O | O | P | E | D | W | I | Y |
| Q | R | R | S | T | U | S | I | N | V |
| W | K | N | I | T | T | I | N | G | X |
| Y | E | T | C | H | I | N | G | Z | A |

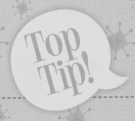

Make a kick chart to keep track of your baby's active and sleepy periods, so you know what is normal for them.

## 117. In other words

Both of you are getting rounder by the minute. Unscramble the anagram:

**TRACKS THERMS**

## 118. Twin up

Keep yourself hydrated. Arrange these ten words into five pairs, each using one word from each box:

| LEMON | MILK | ORANGE | CLUB | WATER |
|-------|------|--------|------|-------|

| SODA | TEA | SHAKE | TONIC | JUICE |
|------|-----|-------|-------|-------|

## 119. Word sandwich

Your pelvis is starting to drift apart. What word inside the parentheses defines both the words outside the parentheses?

**JOINT (___) COOL**

You have passed the halfway mark: You've done the scans and tests, bought the comfy pants, and finished the second batch of puzzles. Here is a recap of the journey so far for you and your baby, plus a slightly easier pregnancy quiz.

* Your baby has almost quadrupled in length since week 12 and weighs in at around 2 lbs. Your baby can hiccup, open and close his or her eyes, and has developed taste buds. He or she can also recognize your voice.

* Your baby is also covered in fine hair (lanugo) and coated with a protective layer of what looks like yogurt (vernix caseosa).

* Your hormones will have settled down and you will be calm enough to begin writing your birth plan, which will change every week.

* Your boobs and feet are much larger.

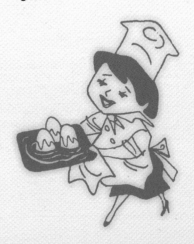

# second trimester pregnancy quiz

1. **How many times bigger than its pre-pregnancy state can the uterus expand?** a) 50  b) 100  c) 500

2. **What causes varicose veins?**
   a) Genes  b) Hormones  c) Weight gain

3. **How much bigger are your feet going to get?**
   a) Under half a size  b) Between half and one size  c) Lady Gargantua

4. **What is the maximum number of weeks at which airlines will allow a pregnant woman to fly?**

5. **Name at least four of the eight B vitamins. Give yourself a bonus for getting them all.**

6. **What are Kegel exercises and how often should you do them?**

7. **Anemia is common in the second trimester. Name six palatable iron-rich foods that can help boost iron in the blood.**

8. **Which of these is not a safe activity when pregnant?**
   a) Pilates  b) Scuba diving  c) Tai chi  d) Yoga

9. **Are stretch marks inevitable on the body? And what percentage of women develop stretch marks?**

10. **Why is it safer to sleep on your left side as your pregnancy advances?**

# third trimester

Well done! You have reached the third trimester, and the end is very nearly in sight, although your feet might not be.

The third trimester (weeks 28–40) is mostly about heartburn, hemorrhoids, and cankles (when calf and ankle join together as one). Your baby is piling on the fat and getting heavier by the minute. By the time you get to the end of this trimester, he or she will have gone from around 2½ lbs. to between 6 and 9 lbs. You probably can't wait to be only carrying your own weight again. It is nature's way of making giving birth seem like the preferable option.

Your brain feels like it is going slower, you get tired easily from hauling yourself, the baby, the placenta, and extra fluid around, and so we have ratcheted the puzzles down even further, and given extra clues to help. The puzzles may not tax the intellect much, but they are designed to entertain and divert you, and get you past the twinges, backache, and other inconveniences. They can be done anywhere, whenever you like.

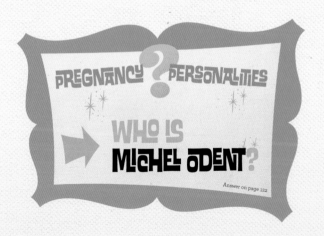

PREGNANCY ? PERSONALITIES

WHO IS MICHEL ODENT?

Answer on page 122

# week twenty-eight

## 120. Quick crossword

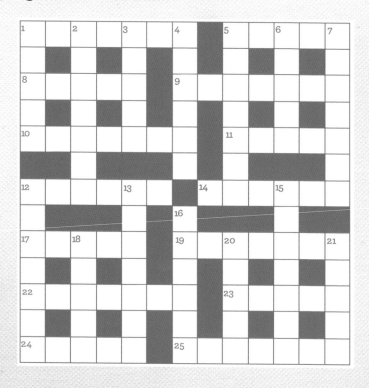

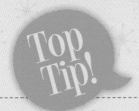

You're in the third trimester; it's getting real. Read up on pain relief and management.

## Across

1. You might choose one of these instead of an OB (7)
5. Delivery of child (5)
8. Goes and shifts (5)
9. Someone who mixes up the elements? (7)
10. Right (7)
11. Molars, incisors etc. (5)
12. Covering for viewers (6)
14. Aided (6)
17. Pleased and satisfied, like a new parent, for example (5)
19. Not the most difficult (7)
22. Beds for babies (7)
23. Splendid (5)
24. Kind of elegance (5)
25. Children's room (7)

## Down

1. To copy (5)
2. End the marriage (7)
3. Edition or topic (5)
4. Stir up (6)
5. Take in air (7)
6. Bring up (5)
7. Came out of an egg (7)
12. Is pregnant (7)
13. Gratify (7)
15. Come before (7)
16. Human being, man, or woman (6)
18. Egg producer (5)
20. Sweet stuff (5)
21. Toy bear (5)

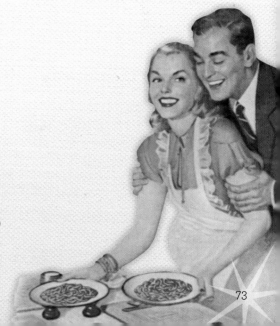

# week twenty-nine

### 121. It all adds up

At this stage your baby weighs around 2½ lbs., which is more or less the same as your brain.

**What is that in terms of 2-oz. chocolate bars?**

### 122. Linked in

What word links these words?

**BATH   DROP   FOLIC   HOUSE   PEEL   TEST**

### 123. In other words

Unscramble the anagram:

**CUE IN MOM**

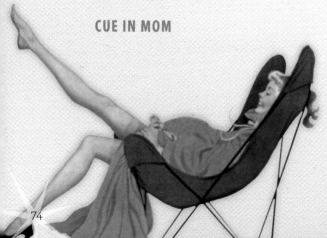

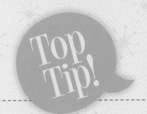

Try to spend as much time as you can with your feet up to prevent swollen ankles.

## 124. Call my bluff

What does "umbilicus" mean?

**BACKACHE**   **LIVE YOGURT**
**INSOMNIA**   **NAVEL**

## 125. Assisted wordsearch

Find the definitions to the clues looking for words that run horizontally, vertically, or diagonally in any direction.

1. Baby transport
2. Receptacle
3. Cloth square
4. Elvis the _ _ _ _ _ _
5. Person who helps with birth
6. Pain relief
7. You haven't seen these in a while

| A | Y | M | C | D | E | F | S |
|---|---|---|---|---|---|---|---|
| J | T | I | I | H | G | E | T |
| K | T | D | L | M | O | Y | R |
| P | O | W | Q | T | S | B | O |
| E | P | I | D | U | R | A | L |
| T | U | F | V | W | S | B | L |
| X | P | E | L | V | I | S | E |
| Y | Z | D | I | A | P | E | R |

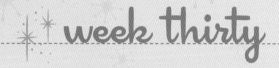

## week thirty

### 126. Word chain

Constipation strikes. Eat more roughage. Can you get from "hard" to "soft" in six smooth moves?

HARD _____ _____ _____ _____ _____ SOFT

### 127. In opposition

Braxton Hicks contractions (practice labor) kick in. What is the opposite of "contraction"?

**DETRACTION**  **EXTRACTION**  **TRACTION**
**EXPANSION**  **ATTRACTION**

### 128. What is not?

Baby's brain is now buzzing with neural networks, unlike yours. Which of these is not part of the brain?

**WHITE MATTER**  **GRAY MATTER**
**DARK MATTER**  **DURA MATER**

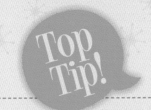
Top Tip!

Shake out your hands and feet to get rid of pins and needles caused by your uterus pressing on blood vessels.

## 129. Word sandwich

Place a word in the parentheses that means the same as the two words outside the parentheses:

**THREAD (_____) BRAN**

## 130. Puzzler

What does this mean?

**L I G A M E N T S**

## 131. Soundalikes

You are feeling quite large now. Below is a trio of definitions that will lead you to words that sound alike but are spelled differently and mean different things.

**SMALL COUNTRY**
**MARINE MAMMALS**
**CRIES OF DISTRESS**

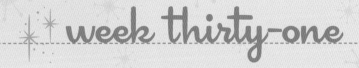

# week thirty-one

## 132. Same old, same old

If you press gently on your belly, your baby may kick back in response. Which word means the same as "answering back exactly"?

RECALIBRATE

RECIPROCATE

REANIMATE

REJUVENATE

REACTIVATE

REGURGITATE

## 133. Twin up

Your baby weighs about 3½ lbs., almost as much as a large stuffed chicken. Pair up these eight words to find four chicken breeds, taking one word from each box:

| BUFF | GIANT | PLYMOUTH | BLUE |
| --- | --- | --- | --- |
| JERSEY | IOWA | ORPINGTON | ROCK |

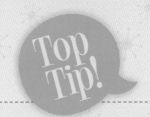
## 134. Word dial

Make as many words as you can of three or more letters, always including the central letter. Give yourself an extra point for making a word out of all the letters.

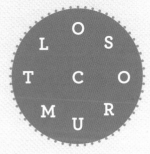

## 135. Word in the middle

What word can be added to the end of the word on the left of the parentheses and the beginning of the word on the right of the parentheses to make two new phrases?

**BIRTHING (_ _ _ _) TABLE**

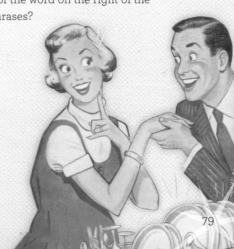

# week thirty-two

### 136. Call my bluff

Your baby can now sleep and dream. Which is the acronym for dream-phase sleep?

RAM    REM    RIM    ROM    RUM

### 137. Enigma variations

Your baby is the size of a smallish melon. Can you crack this code?

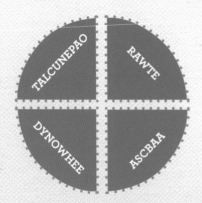

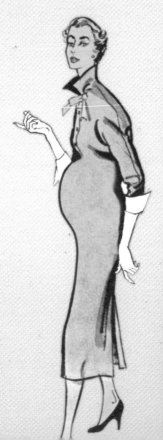

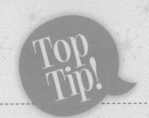

Move over to slip-on shoes, as you won't be able to reach your shoelaces to tie them up.

## 138. Word sandwich

The nesting instinct is kicking in. Place a word in the parentheses that means the same as the two words outside the parentheses:

PUSH ( _ _ _ _ _ ) IRON

## 139. Sort and shift

Your baby is getting short of space in the womb. Sort these six words into two categories:

CAVE  CHAMBER  DEN
HALL  LAIR    ROOM

1
2

# week thirty-three

## 140. Assisted wordsearch

Find the definitions to the clues, looking for words that run horizontally, vertically, or diagonally in any direction.

1. All in one
2. For little feet
3. For little hands
4. For little heads
5. To prevent spills
6. To stay cozy

| T | E | K | N | A | L | B | W |
|---|---|---|---|---|---|---|---|
| A | E | I | S | E | N | O | S |
| T | B | C | D | E | R | F | N |
| E | G | B | H | G | I | J | E |
| N | K | I | Y | L | M | N | T |
| N | O | B | P | V | W | S | T |
| O | A | Q | R | S | T | U | I |
| B | O | O | T | I | E | S | M |

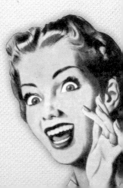

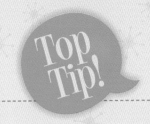

Top Tip!

Start organizing your baby clothes.
Don't underestimate the number
of onesies you will need.

### 141. **Word chain**

You need to keep up omega-3 and iron levels. Can you get from "fish" to "meat" in four servings?

FISH _____ _____ _____ MEAT

### 142. **Odd one out**

Which is the odd word out?

EEL                HERRING          HADDOCK
SALMON          KIPPER           SNAPPER

### 143. **In other words**

Your baby may have regular bouts of hiccups now. Unscramble the anagram:

**A DIM GRAPH**

# week thirty-four

### 144. What is not?

Beans are good for you! Which of these is not, botanically, a bean?

FRENCH BEAN      RUNNER BEAN
LIMA BEAN      KIDNEY BEAN
CHICKPEA      JELLY BEAN

### 145. Word in the middle

Your baby's eyes are working now. What word can be added to the end of the word on the left of the parentheses and the beginning of the word on the right of the parentheses to make two new phrases?

FORE (_____) LINE

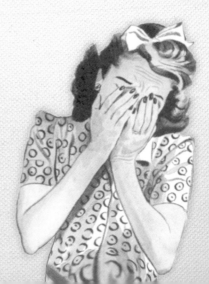

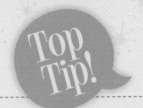

**Top Tip!** Indulge yourself with a manicure and pedicure—nails grow quicker in pregnancy.

## 146. **Word dial**

Your baby is really filling the space now. Make as many words as you can of three or more letters, always including the central letter. Give yourself an extra point for making a word out of all the letters.

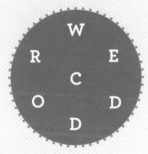

## 147. **Puzzler**

Good news! Nausea is back because of organ crowding. Eat tiny portions, more often, while you solve the puzzler.

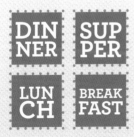

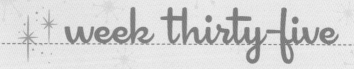

# week thirty-five

### 148. Odd one out

Which of these is not a ring you can wear?

ETERNITY      ENGAGEMENT      WEDDING
SIGNET         MOOD             BENZENE

### 149. Sort and shift

You will need a bag to take your stuff to the hospital. Sort these six words into two categories:

BACKPACK      CARRIER BAG      HOLDALL
OVERNIGHT BAG   RUCKSACK       SUITCASE

1

2

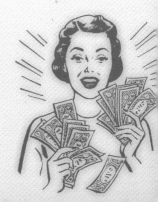

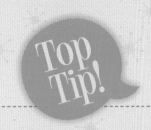

Top Tip!

Take off any tight-fitting rings until after delivery, as your fingers are swelling.

## 150. Enigma variations

You are entering countdown phase. Can you crack this code?

ENO     OWT     EERHT     RUOF     _ _ _ _

## 151. In opposition

The bones of your baby's skull have not yet fused. This allows the head to adjust through the birth canal. What is the opposite of "fused"?

SEPARATE          ELECTRIFIED
REFUSED           EXPLOSIVE

## 152. Same old, same old

Get ready to leave work. Which word, from the Greek, means the same as "to do with work"?

ERGONOMIC        ECONOMIC        GASTRONOMIC
PANORAMIC        ASTRONOMIC      MICROSCOPIC

# week thirty-six

### 153. Call my bluff

Your baby's hiccups may now wake you up at night. What does "onomatopoeia" mean?

A rash on the back of the knees

An obsession with carpets

A word that sounds like what it means

An imaginary state or place where everyone is a yoga master

Irrational fear of Japanese conceptual artists

An ancient branch of geometry

### 154. Word in the middle

What word can be added to the end of the word on the left of the parentheses and the beginning of the word on the right of the parentheses to make two new phrases?

GRAND (_____) SHIP

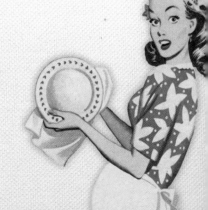

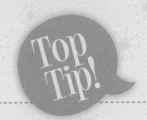

**Top Tip!**

Pack your bag for the hospital, or get things organized for your home birth.

### 155. Word chain

Your baby is developing his or her sucking reflex. Can you get from "suck" to "blow" in eight steps?

SUCK _____ _____ _____ _____ _____ _____ _____ BLOW

### 156. In other words

Your baby's lungs and respiratory system are the last thing to develop. Unscramble the anagram:

**PRAYER RIOTS**

### 157. Word sandwich

You'll be curious about what your baby will look like. Place a word in the parentheses that means the same as the words either side of the parentheses:

WHAT'S INSIDE (_____) SATISFIED

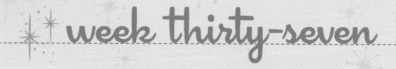

# week thirty-seven

## 158. Odd one out

Time to stock the freezer. Which of the following is not a form of ice-cream treat?

SORBET          GRANITA
SUNDAE         BAKED ALASKA
BOMBE SURPRISE    MONDAE

## 159. Twin up

You probably feel as if you will never have your baby, but are doomed to roam the world the size of two hippos. Organize your e-mail and phone contacts so you are ready to announce the big news. Match these eight words into four pairs, taking one from each box:

| BLACK | ELECTRONIC | I | ADDRESS |
|---|---|---|---|
| PHONE | BOOK | BERRY | MAIL |

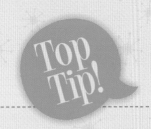

**Top Tip!**

Invest in breast pads; your boobs may be glorious but they may also start to leak colostrum.

### 160. Sort and shift

Goodbye heartburn! Hello constantly full bladder! Sort the following six words into two categories:

ADIOS        CIAO        GOODBYE
FAREWELL    HELLO      WELCOME

1

2

### 161. Soundalikes

Can you find the two words that sound the same but mean something different from the definitions below?

**What you will be giving very soon / bed on a boat**

### 162. What is not?

Your baby is "lightening," shifting down lower in your abdomen. Which of these is not a form of lightning?

BALL        CONCEALED    FORKED
GREASED     BEAD       SHEET

# ✦ week thirty-eight

## 163. Assisted wordsearch

There is no evidence to suggest that playing classical music to your baby will trigger genius, but now's the time to do it. Using the clues, find the composers' last names, looking for words that run horizontally, vertically, or diagonally in any direction.

1. **Franz Joseph H,**
   Austrian (1732-1809)

2. **George Frideric H,**
   German (1685-1759)

3. **Wolfgang Amadeus M,**
   German (1756-91)

4. **Franz L,** Hungarian (1811-86)

5. **Antonio V,**
   Venetian (1678-1741)

6. **Frederic C,** Polish (1810-49)

7. **Gustav H,** English (1874-1934)

8. **Giacomo P,** Italian (1858-1924)

9. **Johann Sebastian B,**
   German (1685-1750)

10. **Edward E,** English (1857-1934)

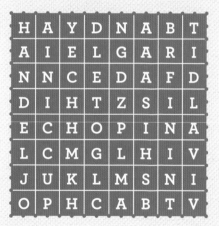

| H | A | Y | D | N | A | B | T |
|---|---|---|---|---|---|---|---|
| A | I | E | L | G | A | R | I |
| N | N | C | E | D | A | F | D |
| D | I | H | T | Z | S | I | L |
| E | C | H | O | P | I | N | A |
| L | C | M | G | L | H | I | V |
| J | U | K | L | M | S | N | I |
| O | P | H | C | A | B | T | V |

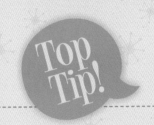

Top Tip!

Hormones can make your eyes dry.
Protect them with "artificial tears"
and sunglasses in bright weather.

### 164. Word in the middle

What word can be added to the end of the word on the left of the
parentheses and the beginning of the word on the right of the
parentheses to make two new phrases?

CONTACT (_____) CAP

### 165. Puzzler

To avoid an ache in your cramped stomach, try six or seven small
snacks rather than three main meals a day. Solve the puzzler.

and and and and and and and and and and and and and and and and and and and and and

### 166. Same old, same old

You may feel you are suddenly far or short-sighted. It will pass. Which
word means the same as "short-sightedness"?

CORNUCOPIA DYSTOPIA MYOPIA
TILAPIA SEPIA UTOPIA

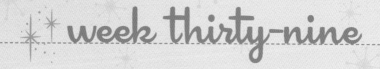

# week thirty-nine

## 167. Sort and shift

Sort the following six words into two categories.

**COCOA**  **COFFEE**  **JUICE**
**MILK**  **TEA**  **WATER**

1

2

## 168. Word sandwich

Your baby's head now has the same circumference as his or her abdomen. Place a word in the parentheses that means the same as the words on either side of the parentheses:

**ROUND (_ _ _ _ _ _ _ _) PUBLICITY LEAFLET**

## 169. In other words

You are clumsier now than when you weren't pregnant, so be careful when washing up. Unscramble the anagram:

**BEFITS GRUNTER**

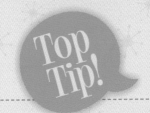

## 170. Call my bluff

Your baby is fully formed and almost ready to appear. What does "vernix caseosa" mean?

A species of Icelandic snail that drinks milk

Specialist varnish used by picture-frame restorers

"Nature's wetsuit," the layer of greasy white stuff your baby is covered in to help him or her slide out more easily

A small town in Umbria

A disease of lactating cows

## 171. Twin up

You may want to redecorate the nursery, again. Don't. Sort these eight words into four pairs instead, taking one from each box.

| BRUSH | PAINT | PAPER | FINISH |
|-------|-------|-------|--------|
| MATTE | GLOSS | SAND | PASTE |

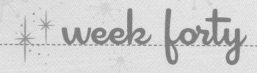

## week forty

### 172. Odd one out

Will it hurt? Which of the following is not a form of pain relief that has been used in childbirth at some point?

**BOTOX**    **CHLOROFORM**    **ENTONOX**
**EPIDURAL**    **PETHIDINE**    **TENS**

### 173. Soundalikes

Your baby will recognize your voice when he or she comes out of the womb. Which words sound the same but fit the different definitions given below?

**AREA OF A WINDOW/AGONY**

### 174. Enigma variations

These numbers will have an important part to play in your very near future. Can you crack the code?

12        1        2        15        18

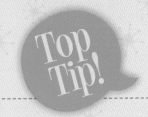

Top Tip!

Nearly there! Stay as active as you can, and keep eating and drinking, although you may not feel like it.

### 175. In opposition

Certain things may get beyond your control. What is the opposite of "incontinent"?

AUSTRALIA     CONTENT     AFRICA
CONSTIPATED     AMERICA     EUROPE
CONTINENT     ASIA

### 176. What comes next?

Think ahead.

P OS TNA T??

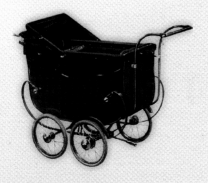

Here we are. You and your baby have put in all the preparation, research and development, and soon it will be the big day. Keep your eyes on the prize. Here is a quick review of your achievements plus an even simpler pregnancy quiz which you don't have to do if you don't feel like it.

* **Your baby is now full term, all systems ready to go; he or she will probably be about 21 inches long and weigh between 6 and 9 lbs. That's about the size of one watermelon.**

* **You may feel a bit more energetic as the baby has dropped farther down into your pelvis, giving you room to breathe and eat.**

* **Your breasts are now glorious, but they and your nipples are tender and you may secrete a yellowish liquid called colostrum.**

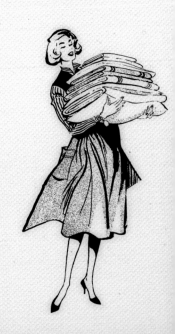

# third trimester pregnancy quiz

1. When should you have gone to prenatal and birthing technique classes?

2. **What initiates labor?**   a) Your hormones   b) The baby's hormones   c) The doctor's schedule

3. How far does your cervix have to open before you can safely start pushing?

4. How long will it take for the cervix to fully dilate?

5. Thinking about pain relief during labor, what is gas and air?

6. What is a mucus plug and where will you find it in the body?

7. What is colostrum and when will your body start producing it?

8. How long will the umbilical cord be when your baby is born?
   a) Roughly 6 inches   b) Roughly 12 inches   c) Roughly 24 inches

9. How many more boys are born than girls (per hundred babies born)?

10. How gorgeous is your baby going to be on a scale of one to ten?

# full term

This is it. Here we are. You must stop pretending that it's all just Braxton Hicks—you will soon have to give birth.

If you have reached 40 weeks, and can make a rough guess at your conception date, you should be ready to give birth any moment now. Your baby is fully formed, ready to thrive outside the womb. Usually, he or she will by now have "dropped," sinking down into the pelvic cradle, which means less heartburn and a restored appetite. This is great because it will help you keep up energy levels for the labor which, as the word makes clear, is hard, but rewarding, work.

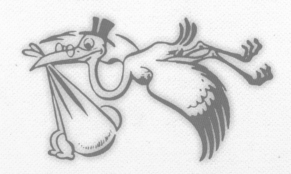

This section is shorter and slightly different as it covers first-stage labor, second-stage labor, birth, and afterwards, plus two pages of puzzles to get you through night feeds. Don't think you don't need these puzzles. Waiting for a cervix to dilate can be pretty tedious stuff and it's good to have something to concentrate on between the contractions. Even in the delivery room, they may be more effective than gas and air, although you might want to ask your birthing partner to hold the book while you shout the answers. Plus, your prize is a gorgeous baby.

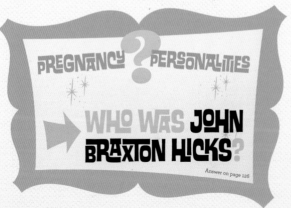

PREGNANCY ? PERSONALITIES

➤ WHO WAS JOHN BRAXTON HICKS?

Answer on page 126

# stage one labor

## 177. In opposition

You are in the early phase of labor. What is the opposite of "early"?

| | | |
|---|---|---|
| LATE | ON TIME | PUNCTUAL |
| TARDY | OVERDUE | I DON'T CARE |

## 178. What comes next?

You may be monitored by high-tech machinery that makes strange noises. What comes next in this sequence?

PANG!    PENG!    PING!    PONG!    _ _ _ _!

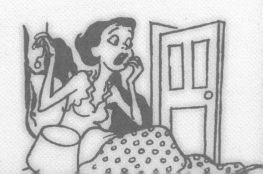

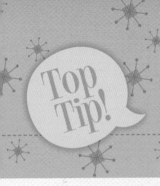

**Top Tip!** Stay calm, and walk when you can. This stage could take hours or even days.

## 179. Enigma variations

Your amniotic sac may break. Can you crack this code?

**WAT ERS**

## 180. Assisted wordsearch

As the contractions bite, think of your favorite things. This assisted wordsearch may help. All the words run left to right horizontally and there are seven of them.

1. small cats
2. children's gloves
3. useful for tying
4. small horses
5. can be rung
6. wintery white stuff
7. good with olives

| K | I | T | T | E | N | S |
|---|---|---|---|---|---|---|
| M | I | T | T | E | N | S |
| S | T | R | I | N | G | A |
| P | O | N | I | E | S | B |
| B | E | L | L | S | C | D |
| S | N | O | W | E | D | G |
| M | A | R | T | I | N | I |

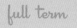

# stage two labor

### 181. Puzzler

It's not all about the uterus. Solve the puzzler.

**EHCA CABK**

### 182. Word in the middle

What word can be added to the end of the word on the left of the parentheses and the beginning of the word on the right of the parentheses to make two new phrases?

**PAIN (_____) MAP**

### 183. Twin up

This is the active phase of labor. Keep your mind active by pairing up these four words, taking one word from each box:

| AGAIN | BIRTH |
|---|---|
| CHILD | NEVER |

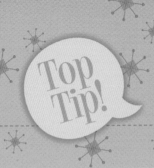

Top Tip!

Take a potty break every hour—your bladder's signals that it is full are no longer reaching you.

### 184. **Word chain**

Your cervix is effacing (getting thinner) and dilating at the same time. Go from "ouch" to "aarg" any way you like.

OUCH _____ _____ _____ _____ AARG

(you may go in one step if you feel like it)

### 185. **What is not?**

Your uterus is transforming from an upside-down pear to a tube rather like a footless sock. Which of the following is not a form of footwear?

SOCK      SHOE      SLIPPER
SANDAL      MULE      SOMBRERO

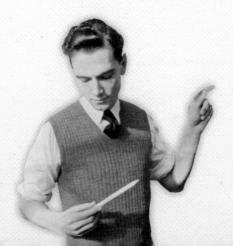

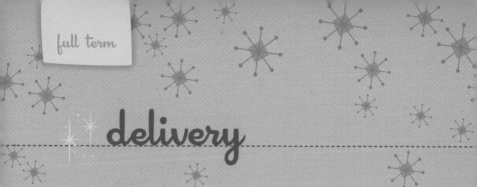

# delivery

## 186. Odd one out

Your baby is now the size of a planet but you are not. Which of these is also not a planet?

| | | |
|---|---|---|
| URANUS | SATURN | MARS |
| JUPITER | VENUS | PLUTO |
| MERCURY | GOOFY | NEPTUNE |

## 187. Mini Crossword

### Across

1. Not cat (3)
3. Not off (2)
5. Not bad (4)

### Down

1. Gets rid of pain (4)
2. Opposite of come (2)
4. Agree without speaking (3)

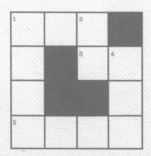

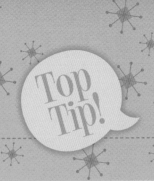

**Top Tip!** Devise a mantra, preferably with a tune, to help you get through the pain peaks.

## 188. **In other words**

Unscramble the anagram:

BBYA

## 189. **Wordplay**

Make as many words as you can, of any kind, from the letters in this word

TRANSITION

## 190. **Rhyme and reason**

Find as many words as you can that:

a) rhyme with

b) mean the same as

BREATHE

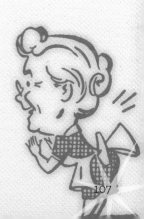

# after the birth

## 191. Find the lady

Your baby will be tested for reflex responses. Which one of these is named after the woman who invented the tests?

APGAR      RADAR      LUNAR
SOLAR      POLAR

## 192. Soundalikes

If you had an episiotomy or a tear, you have stitches. What three words sound the same but fit these definitions?

THEREFORE      PLANT SEED      STITCH

## 193. Linked in

Soon you will be able to see your toes. What links these words?

SPA      FETISH      NOTE
BALL      STEP      BRIDGE
LOOSE      WORK      STOOL

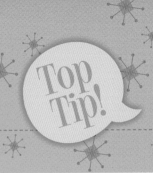

**Top Tip!**

Do not get depressed that your tummy does not go flat instantaneously. It will eventually deflate.

## 194. Call my bluff

You finally get to see your baby. What does "fontanelle" mean?

a medieval love lyric

a small water feature

soft icing for cupcakes

the soft spot on a baby's head where the skull bones haven't yet fused

a very ornate typeface

a minor pantomime character

## 195. In other words

Well done you! Unscramble the anagram. You have three chances at the same word.

NATAL OUTSCORING!

LAGUNO TRACTIONS!

OCARINA GLUTTONS!

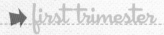 **first trimester**

## Pregnancy Personalities

Fallopius was **Gabriele Falloppio** (*1523–62*), Italian anatomist and physician, who studied the reproductive organs and gave his name to the Fallopian tubes that link the ovaries to the uterus.

# preconception

1. Motion

2. Contraception

3. Onesie: it is the only word without a double consonant

4. You could get around 55 words from the letters in the word "mood swing":

   dingo, disown, dog, doing, domino, don, dong, doom, dosing, dow, down, downs, dowsing,

   gismo, god, godson, goo, good, goods, goon, gown,

   ion, isogon,

   mid, misdo, miso, mod, moo, mood, MOODSWING,

   mooing, moon, mow, mowing, mown,

   nod, now,

   owing, own,

   smog, snow, sod, son, song, soon, sow, sowing, sown, swoon,

   wisdom, won, woo, wood, woods, wooing

5. Vellicate

# week one

6. Floor

7. rattle teddy bricks (toys)
   ball net racket (tennis)
   maraca triangle tambourine (instruments)
   square polygon circle (shapes)

8. RIKK

   This is an anagram of Kirk, captain of the Starship Enterprise; the others are anagrams of famous child doctors

   Richard FERBER, Harvey KARP, William SEARS, Benjamin SPOCK, and Virginia APGAR

9. LADITS

   Like a Diamond in the Sky: the puzzle is made up of the first letter of the lyrics in the first verse and refrain of "Twinkle, Twinkle, Little Star"

   Twinkle twinkle little star
   How I wonder what you are
   Up above the world so high
   Like a diamond in the sky
   Twinkle twinkle little star
   How I wonder what you are

## week two

10. WORM wort wert welt wilt silt SILK

11. You could get around 130 words from the letters in the word "maternity":

    aery, aim, aimer, air, airmen, airy, amen, amenity, amine, amir, amity, anime, ant, ante, anti, any, anytime, are, arm, army, art, arty, ate, attire, aye,

    ear, earn, eat, era, ern, eta,

    imaret, inmate, irate, iterant,

    main, man, mane, many, mar, mare, marine, mart, marten, martin, martinet, mat, mate, MATERNITY, matt, matte, matter, may, mean, meant, meany, meat, meaty, meta, minaret, myna,

    name, namer, nary, nattier, natty, nay, near, neat, nitrate,

    raiment, rain, rainy, ram, ramie, ran, rani, rant, rat, rate, ratite, ratten, ratty, ray, ream, remain, reman, retain, retina, ria,

    taint, tame, tamer, tan, tar, tare, tarn, tart, tarty, tat, tea, team, tear, teary, teat, tenia, terai, tertian, tetany, tetra, tinea, titan, train, trait, tram, tray, treat, treaty, tryma, tyramine, tyrant,

    yam, yamen, yare, yarn, yea, yean, year, yearn, yenta

12. Eructation

13. Uterus

14. Egg

## week three

15. Metal

16. Micturition

17. Taste buds

18. You could get around 45 words from the letters in the word "umbilical":

    abulic, ail, aim, alibi, allium, ami, aulic,

    bacilli, bail, bill, bima, bulimia, bulimiac, bulimic,

    cilia, cilium, claim, climb,

    iamb, iambi, iambic, ilia, iliac, ilial, ilium, ill,

    labium, laic, lib, lilac, lima, limb, limba, limbi, limbic, limuli,

    mail, malic, miaul, mib, mica, milia, mill,

    UMBILICAL, umiac

19. Rapid or excessive blinking

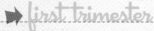

## week four

20. Cat: the extra work your body is putting in makes you tired and you snatch snoozes wherever you can, just like a cat

21. WIND wine pine pane pale palm CALM

22. Fallopian

23.
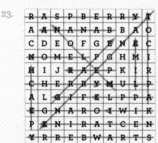

RASPBERRY   ORANGE
BANANA   NECTARINE
LEMON   STRAWBERRY
PEAR   PEACH
PLUM   LIME
CHERRY   APRICOT
APPLE   GRAPE
FIG   TANGERINE
KIWI   MELON

## week five

24. Larkspur Ferdinand

25. Packham: both its vowels are the same

26. cream milk lemon (added to drinks)
chocolate tea coffee (drinks)
jug pot cup (receptacles)
sugar honey molasses (sweeteners)

27. Fuji mitsu

## week six

28.
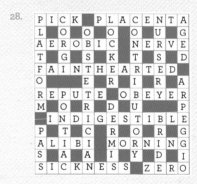

## week seven

29. Tennis coach
    Ball boy
    Second service
    Match point
    Mixed doubles
    Grand slam
    Line judge
    Foot fault

30. The word "the" is repeated

31. Hatch

32. Fireproof

33. Amniotic

## week eight

34. Air/heir
    Beer/bier
    Creak/creek
    Discreet/discrete
    Earn/urn
    Flour/flower

35. Swell

36. Garrulous

37. Tempranillo

## week nine

38.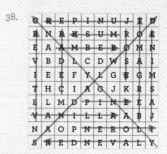

JUNIPER     VETIVER
MUSK        CEDAR
AMBER       ROSE
PINE        BERGAMOT
VANILLA     JASMINE
NEROLI      SANDALWOOD
LAVENDER    YLANGYLANG

39. Air: you can put it in front of each of these words and get another word

40. SCENT stent stint STINK

41. Drip

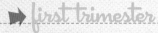 **first trimester**

## week ten

42. Vionnet: Madeleine Vionnet was a Parisian couturier

43. red yellow blue
    (primary colors)
    green purple orange
    (secondary colors)
    red blue purple
    (red + blue = purple)
    yellow red orange
    (yellow + red = orange)
    blue yellow green
    (blue + yellow = green)

44. Solidify

45. Hydration

46. Soporific

## week eleven

47. You could get around 80 words from the letters in the word "epidermis":

    dip, deep, deeps, demirep, deperm, drip,

    empire, emprise, EPIDERMIS, epiderm, epimer, espied,

    imp, imped, impede, impeder, impi, impis, imprese,

    ped, pedes, pee pee, peer, peers, peise, peised, per, peri, perm, permed, perms, perse, pes, pie, pied, pier, piers, pies, pis, pismire, premed, premeds, premie, premies, premise, premised, preside, pride, pried, pries, prim, prime, primed, primi, prims, prism, psi,

    redip, rep, rip, ripe, riped, ripes,

    seep, seer, sempre, simp, simper, simpered, sip, sped, speed, sperm, spider, spied, spier, spiered, spire, spired, spree

48. Mental: all the other words have the vowels *a* and *e* appearing in alphabetical order

49. A sulphur-based water-soluble vitamin of the B complex

50. Amniocentesis

## week twelve

51. Parturition

52. SPIT spot soot loot look lock LICK

53. You could get around 75 words from the letters in the word "flatulent":

    aft, alt, ant, ante, ate, attune, aunt,

    eat, eft, eluant, eta, etna,

    fat, fate, fatten, fault, faun, feat, felt, fet, feta, fetal, flat, flatten, FLATULENT, flaunt, fluent, flute,

    lat, late, laten, latent, latte, latten, leant, left, lent, let, lunate, lunet, lute,

    neat, net, nut, nutate, nutlet,

    tael, tale, talent, tall, tan, tat, tau, taunt, taut, tauten, tea, teal, teat, tel, tela, tell, ten, tent, tet, tufa, tuft, tule, tulle, tun, tuna, tune, tut,

    unfelt, uta

54. Wah: The puzzle is made up of lyrics from the children's song "The Wheels on the Bus"

The wheels on the bus go round and round,

round and round, round and round.

The wheels on the bus go round and round, all through the town.

The wipers on the bus go swish, swish, swish;

swish, swish, swish; swish, swish, swish.

The wipers on the bus go swish, swish, swish, all through the town.

The horn on the bus goes beep, beep, beep;

beep, beep, beep; beep, beep, beep.

The horn on the bus goes beep, beep, beep, all through the town.

The babies on the bus go "wah, wah, wah;

wah, wah, wah; wah, wah, wah."

The babies on the bus go "wah, wah, wah," all through the town.

The mommies on the bus go "shh, shh, shh;

shh, shh, shh; shh, shh, shh."

The mommies on the bus go "shh, shh, shh," all through the town.

55. Medical term for nosebleed

# first trimester pregnancy quiz

1. **A zygote is what is produced when sperm meets and fertilizes egg; an embryo develops after a zygote's cells have multiplied, which takes about 14 days. An embryo becomes a fetus at 8 weeks**

2. **Human chorionic gonadotrophin, or HCG. It is made by the placenta**

3. **Y chromosome, supplied by the male partner**

4. **X chromosome, supplied by the male partner**

5. **It minimizes the occurrence of neural tube defects in your baby**

6. **Between 22 and 28 lbs.**

7. **None until the second trimester according to the National Institutes of Health**

8. **75 percent**

9. **The heart**

10. **At least 2 pints**

## ➤ second trimester
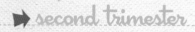

### pregnancy personalities

**Professor Ian Donald** (*1910–87*), Scottish obstetrician, introduced the use of ultrasound scanning in pregnancy in the early 1960s.

# week thirteen

56. **You could get around 65 words from the letters in the word "dentistry":**

    deist, deity, den, density, dent, dentist, DENTISTRY, deny, destiny, dey, die, diet, din, diner, direst, dirt, dirty, distent, dit, dite, ditsy, ditty, driest, dry, driest, dye, dyer,

    end,

    ides, ired,

    nerd, nerdy, nide,

    red, rend, resid, rid, ride, rident rind, rinsed, rynd,

    send, side, sired, sited, snide, snider, strid, stride, strident, syndet,

    tend, tide, tidy, tied, tinder, tindery, tined, tinted, tired, trend, trendy, trident, tried, trysted, tyned

57. **Ulna: it is not an organ, but a bone in the arm**

58. **Tooth**

59. **Drill**

60. **Mouthwash**

# week fourteen

61.

| A | C | U | T | I | C | L | A | B | A |
|---|---|---|---|---|---|---|---|---|---|
| P | O | N | Y | T | A | I | L | K | D |
| A | C | X | E | T | R | O | C | E | N |
| F | A | I | A | L | P | O | I | R | E |
| U | F | D | D | E | L | O | L | A | T |
| R | A | F | N | D | A | P | L | T | I |
| D | H | G | A | H | N | M | O | I | L |
| N | S | E | B | I | U | A | F | N | P |
| A | R | A | O | B | G | H | I | C | S |
| D | P | O | R | C | O | S | B | O | B |

CUTICLE     BAND
PONYTAIL   LANUGO
CORTEX      SHAMPOO
PLAIT       FOLLICLE
CROP        KERATIN
BOB         SPLIT ENDS
DANDRUFF   DREADLOCKS
SHAFT

62. **PILES pales palms BALMS**

63. **Stretch**

## week fifteen

64. door gate hatch (entrances)
    breast wing thigh (poultry cuts)
    portal femoral jugular (veins)

65. Vane/vain/vein

66. Orgasmic bliss

67. WWW (for "wee wee wee"): the
    puzzle is made up of the first letter
    of the lyrics of the nursery rhyme
    "This Little Piggy"

    This little piggy went to market
    This little piggy stayed at home
    This little piggy had roast beef
    This little piggy had none
    And this little piggy went "wee wee
    wee" all the way home.

## week sixteen

68. Three-letter words:

    ace, ado, ape, arc, are, ave, avo, cad,
    cap, car, cod, coo, cop, dap, dev, doc,
    doe, ear, era, oar, oca, ode, ope, ora,
    orc, ore, ova, pad, par, pea, ped, per,
    pod, pro, rad, rap, rec, red, rep, rev,
    roc, rod, roe, vac, var

Four-letter words:

aced, acre, aero, aped, aper, apod,
arco, area, aver, cade, cape, capo,
card, care, carp, cave, cero, coda,
code, coed, coop, cope, cord, core,
cove, crap, crop, dace, dare, dear,
deco, deva, doer, door, dopa, dope,
dorp, dove, drop, odea, odor, oped,
orad, orca, ordo, over, paca, pace,
para, pard, pare, pave, pear, poco,
pood, poor, pore, proa, prod, race,
rape, rave, read, reap, redo, repo, road,
rode, rood, rope, rove, vara, vera

69. E: the letters taken altogether
    make up the phrase "size of a
    planet"

70. Pica

71. Theobromine

72. Heartburn

## week seventeen

73. Middle: they are all boxing weight
    classes

74. Isthmus

75. Yoga: they are all names of poses

76. Deflated

77. Lumbago

78. Lost in space

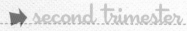 second trimester

## week eighteen

79. Pair/pear/pare
    Or/ore/oar
    Rain/reign/rein
    Ware/where/wear

80. Tibia: it is the only
    one without a *u* in it

81. Group

82. FOOT soot shot SHOE

## week nineteen

83. This is a simple alphabet code—
    replace each letter with the
    previous letter in the alphabet to
    reveal the names:

    Manolo Blahnik
    Christian Louboutin
    Jimmy Choo

84. U: G is the seventh letter of the
    alphabet, N is the fourteenth letter,
    and U is the twenty-first

85. Hide

86. Pollex

87. bran part trap (all have an a)
    Fret lend shed (all have an e)
    Shop most word (all have an o)

## week twenty

88.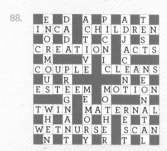

## week twenty-one

89. You could get around 115 words
    from the letters in the word
    "cartwheel":

    ache, aether, arch,

    CARTWHEEL, chalet, char, chare,
    chart, chat, chaw, chawer, cheat,
    cheater, cheer, chela, chelae, chelate,
    chert, chew, chewer, crwth,

    each, earth, eche, etch, etcher, eth,
    ether,

    hale, haler, halt, halter, haltere, hare,
    hat, hate, hater, haw, heal, healer,
    hear, heart, heat, heater, hectare, heel,
    her, here, herl, het, hew, hewer,

    larch, latch, lath, lathe, lather, leach,
    leacher, leather, lech, lecher, leech,
    lehr, letch, lethe,

    rachet, rah, ratch, rath, rathe, reach,
    rechew, reheat, retch, reteach, rhea,

tach, tache, tahr, teach, teacher, thaler, thaw, thawer, the, theca, thecal, thee, there, thew, three, threw,

watch, watcher, wealth, weather, welch, welcher, wether, whale, whaler, what, wheal, wheat, whee, wheel, where, whereat, whet, whew, wrath, wreath, wreathe, wretch

90. Jack in the box

91. In yoga, the pose of the cat

92. Protrude

## week twenty-two

93. Heat

94. Sleep

95. Soft

96. swallow gulp swig (ingestion)
palm nail knuckle (hand)
hawk handsaw rasp (tools)

97. Consistency

## week twenty-three

98. You could get around 35 words from the letters in the word "babybrain":

aba, abba, abri, aby, arb, ayn

baa, baba, baby, BABYBRAIN, ban, bani, bar, barb, barn, barny, bay, bib, bibb, bin, binary, birn, bra, brain, brainy, bran, bray, brin, briny,

nab, nib,

rabbi, rabbin, rib, ribby

99. Ferrum

100. Each half of a pair is an anagram of the other:

Admirer married
Decimal claimed
Large regal
Marines seminar
Night thing

101. MOON morn more mole male tale talk WALK

## week twenty-four

102. Areola

103. Nowhere: they are alive

104. Hemorrhoids

105.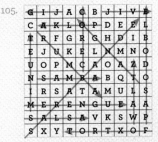

JIG
JIVE
POLKA
SAMBA
MERENGUE
SALSA
FOXTROT

MINUET
CEROC
WALTZ
PASODOBLE
SARABANDE
RUMBA
TANGO

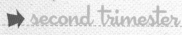 **second trimester**

## week twenty-five

106. Photosynthesis

107. Birth plan

108. Eye

109. CUTSA (for "Climbed Up The Spout Again"): the puzzle is made up of the first letter of the lyrics of the nursery rhyme "The Itsy Bitsy Spider"

   The itsy bitsy spider climbed up the water spout

   Down came the rain, and washed the spider out

   Out came the sun, and dried up all the rain

   And the itsy bitsy spider climbed up the spout again

110. Pound

## week twenty-six

111. You could get around 115 words from the letters in the word "deflation":

   afield, aft, alef, alif, aloft,

   daft, deaf, deal, defat, defi, defiant, DEFLATION, defoliant , deft, delft,

   eft, elf, elfin, enfold,

   fad, fade, fado, fail, failed, fain, faint, fainted, fan, fane, fantod, fat, fate, fated, feat, fed, feint, felid, felon, felt, fen, fend, fet, feta, fetal, fetial, fetid, fiat, fid, fido, fie, field, fiend, fil, fila, file, filed, filet, filo, fin, final, finale, find, fine, fined, fino, fit, flan, flat, flea, fled, flied, flint, flinted, flit, flite, flited, float, floated, floe, flota, foal, foaled, foe, foil, foiled, foined, folate, fold, folia, foliate, foliated, fon, fond, fondle, font, fontal,

   inflate, inflated, infold,

   leaf, left, life, lift, lifted, loaf, loafed, lofted,

   naif, naife, neif,

   oaf, oft, often, olefin,

   tenfold

112. LEFT lift rift rife ride SIDE

113. Side

114. Spinach: it does not have double consonants

115. Blue

## week twenty-seven

116.

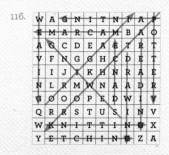

| PAINTING | DRAWING |
|----------|---------|
| MACRAME | READING |
| KNITTING | POTTERY |
| ETCHING | ORIGAMI |
| WEAVING | PATCHWORK |
| DANCE | SEWING |

117. Stretch marks

118. Tonic water
Club soda
Lemon tea
Orange juice
Milk shake

119. Hip

## second trimester pregnancy quiz

1. c) 500

2. Any of these in any combination can cause varicose veins

3. b) between half and one size

4. It depends on the airline, but some say 36 weeks

5. Thiamine, riboflavin, niacin, pantothenic acid, pyridoxine, folic acid, vitamin B12, biotin

6. Kegel exercises strengthen the pelvic floor muscles. As no one can see what you are up to, do them whenever you can

7. Iron-rich foods include: red meat, sardines, beans, eggs, molasses, cashew nuts, whole grain bread, sesame seeds, dark green leafy vegetables, clams, dried fruit, dark chocolate

8. b) Scuba diving

9. No, but very likely; 90 percent, according to Yale University

10. Because the major blood vessels (vena cava and aorta) run down the right side of the spine, and if they get squashed while you sleep, your blood may not flow efficiently

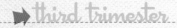

## third trimester

### pregnancy personalities

**Dr. Michel Odent** (b. *1930*), French specialist in maternity and childbirth, pioneered the use of the birthing pool in the 1970s.

## week twenty-eight

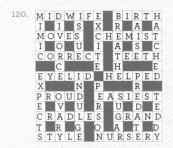

120.

| M | I | D | W | I | F | E |   | B | I | R | T | H |
|---|---|---|---|---|---|---|---|---|---|---|---|---|
| I |   | I |   | S |   | X |   | R |   | A |   | A |
| M | O | V | E | S |   | C | H | E | M | I | S | T |
| I |   | O |   | U |   | I |   | A |   | S |   | C |
| C | O | R | R | E | C | T |   | T | E | E | T | H |
|   |   | C |   | E |   | H |   | H |   |   |   | E |
| E | Y | E | L | I | D |   | H | E | L | P | E | D |
| X |   |   |   | N |   | P |   | R |   |   |   |   |
| P | R | O | U | D |   | E | A | S | I | E | S | T |
| E |   | V |   | U |   | R |   | U |   | D |   | E |
| C | R | A | D | L | E | S |   | G | R | A | N | D |
| T |   | R |   | G |   | O |   | A |   | T |   | D |
| S | T | Y | L | E |   | N | U | R | S | E | R | Y |

## week twenty-nine

121. 20 chocolate bars

122. Acid

123. Meconium

124. Navel

125.

| A | M | M | C | D | E | F | S |
|---|---|---|---|---|---|---|---|
| J | T | I | I | H | G | E | T |
| K | T | D | L | M | O | Y | R |
| P | O | W | Q | T | S | B | O |
| E | P | I | D | U | R | A | L |
| T | U | F | V | W | S | B | L |
| X | P | E | L | V | I | S | E |
| Y | Z | D | I | A | P | E | R |

STROLLER    MIDWIFE
POTTY    EPIDURAL
DIAPER    TOES
PELVIS

## week thirty

126. HARD bard bare bore sore sort SOFT

127. Expansion

128. Dark matter

129. Fiber

130. Stretched ligaments

131. Wales/whales/wails

# week thirty-one

132. Reciprocate

133. Buff Orpington
Jersey Giant
Iowa Blue
Plymouth Rock

134. You could get around 45 words
from the letters in the word
"colostrum":

cloot, clot, clots, clout, col, color,
COLOSTRUM, colt, comous, coo,
cool, coot, cor, corm, cos, cost, cot,
court, crus, crool, crust, culm, cult,
curl, curst, curt, custom, cut,

loco, locum, locus, locust,

moco, mucor, mucro, mulct,

orc,

roc,

scoot, scot, scour, scout, scrotum,
scum, scut

135. Pool

# week thirty-two

136. REM (Rapid Eye Movement)

137. They are all varieties of melon:
water, casaba, cantaloupe, and
honeydew

138. Press

139. cave den lair (all animal spaces)
room hall chamber (all human
spaces)

# week thirty-three

140.

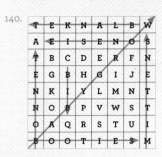

| | | | | | | | |
|---|---|---|---|---|---|---|---|
| T | E | K | N | A | L | B | W |
| A | E | I | S | E | N | O | S |
| T | B | C | D | E | R | F | N |
| E | G | B | H | I | J | E |
| N | K | I | L | M | N | T |
| N | O | B | P | V | W | S | T |
| O | A | Q | R | S | T | U | I |
| B | O | O | T | I | E | S | M |

ONESIE    BONNET
BOOTIES    BIB
MITTENS    BLANKET

141. FISH fist fest feat MEAT

142. Salmon: it does not have double
consonants or vowels

143. Diaphragm

# week thirty-four

144. Jelly bean

145. Sight

146. You could get around
25 words from the letters
in the word "crowded":

cod, codder, code, coded, coder, coed,
cor, cord, corded, core, cored, cow,
cowed, cower, credo, crew, crow,
crowd, CROWDED, crowed,

deco, décor, doc,

orc,

rec

147. Four square meals

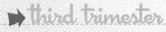

## third trimester

## week thirty-five

148. Benzene

149. suitcase overnight bag carrier bag
(all have four vowels)
rucksack backpack holdall
(all with two vowels)

150. EVIF: the words are the first five
whole numbers spelled backwards

151. Separate

152. Ergonomic

## week thirty-six

153. A word that sounds like what it
means

154. Mother

155. SUCK buck bock book boot soot
slot slow BLOW

156. Respiratory

157. Content

## week thirty-seven

158. Mondae

159. Blackberry
iPhone
Electronic mail
Address book

160. adios ciao welcome
(they don't have any double letters)
hello goodbye farewell
(they have double letters)

161. Birth/berth

162. Concealed

## week thirty-eight

163.

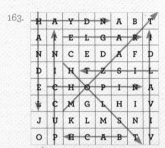

HAYDN    CHOPIN
HANDEL   HOLST
MOZART   PUCCINI
LISZT     BACH
VIVALDI   ELGAR

164. Lens

165. Little and often

166. Myopia

## week thirty-nine

167. cocoa juice tea
(they all have two different vowels
appearing next to each other)
coffee milk water
(none of them have two different
vowels appearing next to each
other)

168. Circular

169. Butterfingers

170. "Nature's wetsuit," the layer of
greasy white stuff your baby is
covered in to help him or her slide
out more easily

171. Paste brush
     Matte finish
     Gloss paint
     Sand paper

## week forty

172. Botox

173. Pane/pain

174. Labor: the numbers stand for letters of alphabet

175. Continent

176. AL: the word is "postnatal"

# third trimester pregnancy quiz

1. Between 34 and 36 weeks, but it's not too late to squeeze in some basic breathing and relaxation techniques

2. b) Hormones from your baby start the labor process by sending messages to the placenta to produce more estrogen and less progesterone, both of which get labor underway

3. 4 inches—about the width of your hand

4. Estimate 1 cm. (under ½ inch) an hour for a first baby, 1.5 cm. (slightly over ½ inch) per hour for subsequent ones

5. Gas and air, or entonox, is a mixture of 50 percent oxygen and 50 percent nitrous oxide, or laughing gas. You can control it yourself and it takes the edge off contractions

6. A mucus plug is a thick "cork" of mucus that blocks the mouth of the cervix until it is time to give birth, when it falls out as the cervix dilates

7. Colostrum is an amber liquid secreted by your breasts just before and for a few days after birth. It is high in fat, protein, and antibodies, and is good for your baby's health, even if you do not intend to breastfeed

8. c) Roughly 24 inches

9. 51 percent boys, 49 percent girls

10. **11**

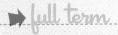

## pregnancy personalities

**John Braxton Hicks** (*1823–97*), English obstetrician, who in 1872 was the first to describe the "practice" contractions now named after him.

# stage one labor

177. Late

178. PUNG: they each have a different vowel

179. Broken waters

180.

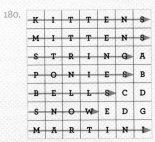

| KITTENS | BELLS |
| MITTENS | SNOW |
| STRING | MARTINI |
| PONIES | |

# stage two labor

181. Back ache

182. Relief

183. Child birth
Never again

184. Our solution is as follows, but you may find yourself uttering other sounds:
OUCH Ourh Oarh Oarg AARG

185. Sombrero

# delivery

186. Goofy (and Pluto for an extra point, as this has now been declassified)

187.

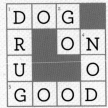

188. Baby

189. You could get around 255 words from the letters in the word "transition":

ai, ains, air, airn, airns, airs, ais, an, ani, anion, anions, anis, anoint, anoints, anon, ant, anti, antiriot, antis, ants, aorist, ar, ariosi, aroint, aroints, ars, arsino, arson, art, artist, arts, as, astir, at, attorn, attorns,

in, inion, inn, inns, ins, instant, instar,
inti, intis, into, intort, intorts, intrant,
intrants, intro, introit, introits, intron,
introns, intros, ion, ions, iota, iotas,
iris, iron, ironist, irons, is, it, its,

na, naoi, naos, naris, nasion, nation,
nations, natron, natrons, nisi, nit,
niton, nitons, nitration, nitrations,
nitro, nitros, nits, no, nona, nonas,
nor, noria, norias, nos, not, nota,

oar, oars, oast, oat, oats, on, onanist,
ons, or, ora, ornis, ors, ort, orts, os,
osar, ostia, otitis, ottar, ottars,

rain, rains, raisin, ran, rani, ranis,
rant, rants, ras, rat, ratio, ration,
rations, ratios, rats, ria, riant, rias,
riot, riots, roan, roans, roast, rosin, rot,
rots, saint, santir, sari, sarin, sat, sati,
satin, satori, si, sin, sir, sit, sitar, snit,
snort, snot, so, soar, son, sonant,
sonar, sora, sori, sort, sot, sri, stain,
stair, star, start, stat, station, stator,
stint, stir, stoa, stoat, strain, strait,
strati, stria, striation, strontia,

ta, tain, tains, taint, taints, tan, tanist,
tans, tanto, tao, taos, tar, tarn, tarns,
taro, taros, tarot, tarots, tars, tarsi,
tart, tarts, tas, tat, tats, ti, tin, tins, tint,
tints, tiro, tiros, tis, tit, titan, titans,
titi, titian, titians, titis, tits, to, toast,
ton, tons, tor, tora, toras, tori, torii,
torn, tors, torsi, tort, torts, tost, tot,
tots, train, trains, trait, traits, trans,
transit, TRANSITION, trio, trios,
triton, tritons, trois, trona, tronas, trot,
trots, tsar

190. Rhymes: seethe, sheathe, teethe,
wreathe
Means the same as: inhale, exhale,
expel, respire

# after the birth

191. Apgar; named for Dr. Virginia
Apgar

192. So/sow/sew

193. Foot

194. The soft spot on a baby's head
where the skull bones haven't
yet fused

195. Congratulations!

## Selected Titles from Seal Press

***The Sh!t No One Tells You: A 52-Week Guide to Surviving Your Baby's First Year***, by Dawn Dais. $16.00, 978-1-58005-484-3. A humorous, realistic, and supportive guide to the first 52 weeks with a baby by best-selling humor author—and new mother—Dawn Dais.

***Bringing in Finn: An Extraordinary Surrogacy Story,*** by Sara Connell. $24.00, 978-1-58005-410-2. A remarkable, moving story of one woman's hard-fought, often painful, journey to motherhood—and the surrogacy experience that changed her family's life.

***The Quarter-Acre Farm: How I Kept the Patio, Lost the Lawn, and Fed My Family for a Year,*** by Spring Warren. $16.95, 978-1-58005-340-2. Spring Warren's warm, witty, beautifully-illustrated account of deciding—despite all resistance— to get her hands dirty, create a garden in her suburban yard, and grow 75 percent of all the food her family consumed for one year.

***Deliver This! Make the Childbirth Choice That's Right for You . . . No Matter What Everyone Else Thinks***, by Marisa Cohen. $14.95, 978-1-58005-153-8. A smart, informative book that helps expectant mothers explore traditional and alternative birthing choices.

***Stay at Home Survival Guide: Field-Tested Strategies for Staying Smart, Sane, and Connected When You're Raising Kids at Home,*** by Melissa Stanton. $15.95, 978-1-58005-247-4. The essential how-to book for stay-at-home mothers, written by a media-savvy former "working mom."

***Beautiful You: A Daily Guide to Radical Self-Acceptance,*** by Rosie Molinary. $16.95, 978-1-58005-331-0. A practical, accessible, day-by-day guide to redefining beauty and building lasting self-esteem from body expert Rosie Molinary.

Find Seal Press Online
www.SealPress.com
www.Facebook.com/SealPress
Twitter: @SealPress